When You Got to Go, You Got to Go

Guide for Emergency Bathroom Use, Bathroom Etiquette & Survival

J. Randal

Copyright © 2021 J. Randal

ALL RIGHTS RESERVED. This book contains material protected under International and Federal Copyright Laws and Treaties. Any unauthorized reprint or use of this material is prohibited. No part of this book may be reproduced or transmitted in any form or by any means, electronic or mechanical, including photocopying, recording, or by any information storage and retrieval system without express written permission from the author/publisher.

Preface

I know how painful it can be when you must go to the bathroom so bad, and there is no place to go. I've suffered from irritable bowel syndrome (IBS) my entire life, so this is a subject with which I am very familiar. I typically use the bathroom six to eight times per day. So, you can imagine how difficult it is for someone like me to maintain a normal life, knowing when I leave the house, a toilet may not be available. I shared a few stories of my struggles in this guide. Some of the stories may be funny to you, but not so much to me. Some stories you will most definitely relate to. I bet many of you experienced much worse conditions. I also shared some personal adventures; not sure why, but I just did.

Regardless of who you are, "When you got to go, you got to go!!!" I wrote this guide hoping I will help some of you deal with this unpredictable bodily function more open-mindedly. Trust me, when you realize your day-to-day mission can be easier and less painful, life will be so much better.

I hope this guide helps you understand not to let this condition dominate you. Plan A is always the number one choice. Plan B, C, D, etc., are also all good choices. Any choice you make will be a good one as long as it's out of your body immediately so you can be on your way.

Table of Contents

- Preface ... iii
- Introduction & Disclaimer ... vi
- Chapter 1:   About my Ventures ... 1
- Chapter 2:   Food ... 6
- Chapter 3:   Public Bathrooms ... 13
- Chapter 4:   Procedures for Safe Bathroom Use ... 18
- Chapter 5:   On the Road & Outside ... 26
- Chapter 6:   Jiffy Johns ... 30
- Chapter 7:   At the Beach ... 35
- Chapter 8:   On a Boat ... 43
- Chapter 9:   Drop & Go ... 49
- Chapter 10: Portable Bathrooms ... 52
- Chapter 11: Closing Remarks ... 55

Introduction

Going to the bathroom is the most unpredictable bodily function every human being has to deal with. It is not a timed or scheduled event. When it is time to go, you have no choice but to go. You can't fight it, and eventually, at some point, it's coming out with or without your permission. You can be stubborn, make this a messy event, or give in and take care of business calmly, safely, and immediately.

This guide outlines many creative places to go to the bathroom and how to protect yourself when you are vulnerable to the surroundings you are forced to endure. Having to go #1 (*urinating*) is much easier for men than women. Men can go anywhere. Most women need shelter, especially when having to go #2 (*poop*). The contents of this guide generally discuss having to go #2 because this is the worst-case scenario for both men and women. However, women could learn how to make #1 much easier if they opened their minds to less attractive, less ladylike alternatives.

If you believe in the Bible, Adam and Eve didn't have bathrooms. They went any place they wanted. I am assuming they buried it. Well, you would hope they did. Today we as human beings have to also think along those lines and not be so proper and sophisticated about this process.

Whoever you are, regardless of how much money or power you have, this process can never be made elegant. It is a gross bodily function every human being experiences, regardless of who you are. It all comes out the same, not in gold or silver or smelling like roses, but a smelly, disgusting mess in whatever consistency it chooses to expel from your body. Do not make your friends or family drive all over creation to find a bathroom for you to use. Use the easy and less painful approach. Be smart about it.

Using public bathrooms can be a living nightmare, especially when you suffer from IBS. I use the bathroom roughly six to eight times daily, sometimes more often on bad days. The only predictable time is first thing in the morning. All other times will happen with little to no notice. It would be an extremely embarrassing situation if you had to leave a business meeting, movie theater, first date, or family gathering so abruptly to make it to the bathroom in time. Could you imagine getting married standing on the altar in front of family and friends, completely nervous, sweating immensely? That time comes demanding attention, and you have seconds to respond. What would you do? You have two choices: blowing in your pants or running to the bathroom. Running to the bathroom is the only sound choice. After you are married, you will be partying with all your friends and family. Hard to do that with a pile of doody in your pants. If this happened to me, I would whisper my dilemma to my soon-to-be wife, not waiting for her permission, and immediately and calmly walk off the stage right towards the bathroom. It could be much worse if the wedding was outside and had you to use a Jiffy John. I hope you are marrying someone with compassion and a sense of humor.

Have you ever walked into the bathroom with only one stall and someone inside who was having a bad day? Well, that happens to me all the time. There are so many variables you have to consider when you plan your bathroom trip. This guide will be addressing many of those variables, including proper etiquette in using public bathrooms to avoid potential germs and diseases.

Depending on your day-to-day schedule, I will discuss items you should consider having on your people, like a flashlight, toilet paper, antibacterial wipes, hand sanitizer, a poop bag, a short camping shovel, and a portable toilet seat. I like to use the Cleanwaste WAG BAG®- GO Anywhere Toilet Kit® biodegradable bags. They are lightweight, Ziplock protected, and puncture-resistant. Each bag contains odor neutralizers and will turn up to 32 ounces of liquids into a solid. You can use this bag for multiple apparatuses. Best of all, they are environmentally friendly and landfill approved. Cleanwaste also has a portable Go Anywhere toilet apparatus seat that folds up into a carrying case. Lightweight, easy to use, and store inside your vehicle. But, it will start to smell in a couple of hours so throw it in the trash can as fast as you can.

When in someone else's vehicle or on foot, you may not have the travel essentials you need to carry with you. Create a bag using a knapsack. You can put in it the important toilet essentials you need and include bottled water, snacks, a change of underwear (*just in case*), and other stuff you may need. The Cleanwaste WAG BAG®- GO Anywhere Toilet Kit® is nice to have in your bag. The bags come with toilet paper and hand sanitizing wipes. You better put some more toilet paper in your bag, as Cleanwaste provides toilet paper for two or maybe three wipes. Try not to overstuff your bag. The heavier the bag, the more difficult it will be to travel with it.

Remember what you eat the night before or during the day plays a huge role, so be smart and plan. I hope this guide will be useful to you in whatever number nature is calling you.

Disclaimer: This guide is designed to provide helpful information on the subjects discussed. Subjects include dealing with uncontrollable urges in having to go to the bathroom when you're away from home or in a public area, options or methods to safely urinate or defecate in emergencies when making it to a suitable public bathroom is unreachable. It is illegal to urinate or defecate willfully in any public area or place not designed for that use. If you choose this illegal act, you will be held responsible for your actions. You may be arrested for some crimes such as indecent exposure, disorderly conduct, or public lewdness. If you have no choice but to assume that risk, it is advised to shield yourself from public sight to the best of your abilities and remove whatever was expelled from your body and take it with you.

This guide is also not meant to be used, nor should it be used to diagnose or treat any medical condition. Some conclusions or stated facts or opinions within this guild were researched on the internet. It is assumed information collected on the internet was accurate and factual.

For diagnosis or treatment of any medical problem, consult your physician. The publisher and author of this guide are not responsible for a person or persons acting irresponsibly. Additionally, the publisher and author of this guide are not responsible for any specific health or allergy needs that may require medical supervision. They are not liable for any damages or negative consequences from any treatment, action, application, or preparation to any person reading or following the information in this book.

References are provided for informational purposes only and do not constitute an endorsement of any illegal act or product. The person or persons reading this guide will be fully responsible for their actions under penalty of law.

1 About My Ventures

I want to share my early life, hoping you can understand why I wrote this guide. I can't tell you how many times I was sitting on the toilet in severe pain, evaluating how to clean up after myself because I soiled my pants and destroyed the bathroom. Like everyone else, I waited to use a normal bathroom. For years I was rushing to find a suitable bathroom while holding it in as best as possible. The pain and suffering I experienced over the past decades were unbearable and unnecessary. Everyone needs to know there are other options to consider.

Most people don't understand exactly how difficult it can be for people who suffer from IBS. There are many forms of IBS. All forms suck, but some require a bathroom at every corner. The IBS disease I suffer from produces explosive diarrhea with significant pain intensified by frustration, stress, and anxiety. Frustration, stress, and anxiety are normal parts of your day-to-day activity. The best job for people like me is a desk job at an office building with bathrooms. The ones reading this guide right now who happen to suffer from IBS know exactly what I'm talking about. When it comes to the pain, you don't have to suffer from IBS to feel what I am talking about. Pain is Pain!!! Soiling your pants or destroying a bathroom is embarrassing and traumatizing, depending on the circumstance. Most all of this can be avoided as long as you take care of yourself.

The personal stories I am about to share with you throughout this guide happened before 1978 when picking up dog poop became mandatory in most states. I always picked up my toilet paper, but it didn't dawn on me to also pick up my poop. When I realized I needed to be more civilized about the process, I started picking up after myself. It was a disgusting, smelly, and intense process that sucked, but I had no choice. It was the right thing to do every time, regardless of where I was. After a while, this became a daily life experience. Over time I became more careful and found many other ways to pick up after myself. Each day I was getting better and better at it. Nowadays, technology has so many portable products and devices you can use. Just search "portable bathrooms" on the internet, and you will see many manufacturers with several products to choose from.

I have one to two close calls per day. Most of the time, I plan my day knowing where all the bathrooms are located. I believe my ass has a mind of its own. When it is time to go, regardless of having a good or bad day, sometimes my ass gets impatient and explodes prematurely when relief is in sight. There must be a direct network between my ass and my eyes. Has anyone else experienced this? I know this sounds crazy, but for some reason, when my eyes see that toilet, I go into an automatic mode with no control of the timing. The only action I have control of is positioning my ass over the drop zone with a 3- to a 6-second window.

I am sure everyone knows what the tripod position is. Tripod is when you plant your two feet on the ground and place your right or left hand on the wall behind you to hover over the toilet, keeping your ass cheeks above the seat. No one wants to sit on a toilet seat without proper recon and protection. We IBS people experience this feeling several times a day. We do not have much choice in finding a clean or suitable bathroom. Sitting on the toilet seat is optional but sometimes necessary, regardless if you have protection or not. We IBS people are grateful to find any place we can call a bathroom.

In my early years, I had to learn really fast about properly using a public bathroom. I didn't fully understand the cleanliness of the bathrooms until I was well into my 30s. As a kid, everywhere my mother took us, I was scouting for bathrooms. I remember being at Playland Amusement Park in Ocean City, Maryland (between 1965 to 1975). My brothers and sisters teased that the bathroom was my favorite ride. Well, they were correct because it seemed I was always riding the toilet more than the amusement rides. My favorite ride was the Monster Mouse, probably the most dangerous ride ever. I believe that ride still exists somewhere. I did leave a surprise on the ride seat a couple of times. My mother had to take me back to the place we stayed at least one time per vacation. I always felt horrible for my brothers and sisters having to deal with me.

When I was in the 9th grade, my class took a field trip to New York City by train. We visited the World Trade Center, Empire State Building, United Nations, not sure what else. I remember walking on the streets of New York on our way to the United Nations Visitors Center, and I had to go to the bathroom so bad I could almost taste it. Okay, that was gross, but you get the picture. Being on the streets of New York City, any establishment with a public bathroom would be a 10- or 20-minute wait at the minimum. There was also a long line to get into the Visitors Center. There was no way I was going to make it. I started scanning the area for places to go. The only place I could find was very risky. I mean verrrrrry risky!!! There were tall bushes in front of the United Nations Visitors Center between the main road and driveway. I found my place and stood right in front, ready to go. I let everyone in my class get in front of me and scanned the area again to see if there were any police or anyone else who may pay attention to me. It then dawned on me I was in New York City. No one cared what I was doing. As long as I was not disturbing their way of life, they could care less. It was definitely a drop-and-run mission. Drop-and-run is when you have no time to plan and no time for a cover.

Drop and run as fast as humanly possible. We talk more about drop-and-runs later in this guide. So, I balled up a big piece of toilet paper and placed it in my front pocket to get ready. As soon as the last kid in my class walked past me, I quickly ducked into the bushes, frantically pulled my pants down, bent over, dropped the load, placed the balled up toilet paper between my ass cheeks, pulled up my pants, and was back on the street in seconds. As soon as I ducked out of the bushes, I ran to catch up with everyone. That was one of the fastest bathroom missions I have ever accomplished, just under eight seconds. I doubt very seriously anyone paid any attention to what I was doing. Once I got into the Visitors Center, I went to the bathroom to finish cleaning up. No issues to report. I got lucky; it was a clean getaway.

For those who do not know what a clean getaway is, you go #2, and the poop is so firm it does not leave a mark; therefore, wiping is unnecessary. In cases when you experience a clean getaway, you still need to use a checker. The checker is at least one toilet paper wipe to be sure you have no marks. If you believe you experienced a clean getaway, don't be bold and assume all is good. Trust me; the chances are you have marks. I would say one out of ten clean getaways are mark-free. Not good odds. So, if I were you, I would always use a checker.

Shortly after high school, I was in a bad place. I was always drunk off my ass, angry, dead-end job, no money, completely lost. I was an asshole and a loser. There was no place for me in this world. When I was 19 years old, I enlisted in the Army. Not the best job to have when you suffered from IBS, but there were no other options at the time. I can honestly say the Army saved my life and made me a better person.

The most embarrassing Army moment for me was towards the end of advanced individual training (AIT). I was on my way back from the mess hall in formation. I asked the drill sergeant if I could pull out of formation to run to the barracks so I could use the bathroom. After we exchanged words about me being a pussycat, I started running towards the barracks. I had to stop at least five times to fight through the pain. I was determined not to explode in my pants, so I kept on fighting. Once I got to the barracks, I was about ten feet away from the bathroom door when a woman second lieutenant, just out of the academy, stopped me in the hallway and ordered me to stand at attention, dictating to me about my "duty" in respecting officers.

There I stood in severe pain, sweating as she started disciplining me in a stern, loud voice. I was so pissed and angry while she was drilling her finger into my chest and spewing her stinking breath. Jesus Christ, it was horrible. Like being sprayed in the mouth by a skunk while eating monkey-shit and washing it down with spoiled milk. Yeah, you get the picture. So, I fought back using the human version of Agent Orange and exploded right in front of her while standing at attention. It was loud, nasty-smelling, and abundant with liquid running out of my pant legs onto the floor surrounding her. The look on her face was priceless. She was so grossed out and shocked that this was really happening. I looked right into her eyes and said, *"I guess we both learned something this morning."* I never ran into her again after that day. I believe she transferred to another platoon or company. She may have won the battle being an officer, but I won the war!!! She received exactly what she was demanding from me. Good riddance. She was a bitch anyway.

Over the years, I've always tried to be prepared before leaving the house. I pack a flashlight, toilet paper, hand sanitizer, portable toilet seat, a large cup, and poop bags. Again, I like using Cleanwaste WAG BAG®- GO Anywhere Toilet Kit® portable, biodegradable bags. In my opinion, they are perfect. Poop in one bag, place in another Ziplock bag and throw it away. You can carry the loaded bag inside your vehicle for an hour or two before it starts to smell.

You never know when that special feeling will arise again. Whenever you're away from home, always be prepared!!!

2 FOOD

Most of us have busy lives, and being on the road is part of the workday. No one can predict road conditions, much less the weather. Chances are you will have a bad experience and not make it to the toilet in time. It may happen more times than you like to admit. There are ways to limit those bad experiences, but you have to stand strong and make changes in your life. The first step is to try and defend yourself from emergency bathroom use. We all heard this statement, "*You are what you eat.*" Now think of the reality of that statement, "*What goes in must come out!*" So be careful in what you eat or drink the night before and especially when you're on the road. Be careful of sugar substitutes, fatty foods, fiber, dairy and spicy foods, to name a few. Overeating will quickly put you on the toilet. You know yourself better than anyone does. If you know what food causes you problems, don't eat those foods the night before or during the day.

You have the power to turn a potentially disastrous emergency into a planned bathroom experience. All you need to do is be smart about what food you eat, who you buy it from, and how much you consume. All of these factors are extremely important. I'm not a doctor or nutritionist, but what I am discussing is common sense. Just because you add lettuce to a sandwich does not make it a healthy choice. There are so many things to think about before you eat.

The best solution is to prepare your food at home the night before, regardless of where you are going. Some will say, "*I don't have time to make my lunch,*" rambling on listing countless reasons why they don't have the time—what a lazy statement. Everyone has time to prepare food the night before. You find time to take a shower, watch TV, read the paper, go to the bathroom, do laundry, have sex. Normal life dictates all of us having to do many common activities every day. Preparing food for the following day would be considered one of those day-to-day activities. Just fit it into your schedule. Turn off the TV and make a sandwich.

Even if you're good about preparing food for the following day, there are always unpredictable circumstances requiring you to eat on the run. Yep, those days happen more than you realize. We all know fast food joints may not be the best choice. But when you're hungry, you have to eat. While you're looking for a place to eat, you should think more along the fuel lines and not what is nutritionally good for you. In every case, before you choose what to eat, ask yourself this question, "*Will this food put me on the toilet*?" You have to be smart in the food place you choose and what you choose to eat.

I have a system I would like to share with you. It works for me, and I believe it will work for you as long as you stick to it. Consider the following steps when you have no choice but to eat away from home.

- We know it's important to stay hydrated, but be smart in how much liquid you consume before starting your day. Most of us need our coffee in the morning and will most likely drink it on the way to work. Try to limit yourself to 8 ounces of coffee to get your eyes open and alert.
  When you reach your destination, drink all the coffee you want. I love coffee a lot. I have to drink decaffeinated because caffeine gives me diarrhea and makes my heart flutter. On the way to work, I stop for a large 20-ounce coffee. I use an insulated cup, so my coffee stays hot for a long time. When I am close to my destination, I start

drinking my coffee. This works out perfectly for me. Shortly after my destination is reached, it's time to drain it all out.

- You have to remember the golden rule. <u>NEVER</u> chose a restaurant that prepares your food with their bare hands. Trust me; their hands are not clean. I don't care if they use a grinder soaked in alcohol. I don't want any of those people making me a sandwich. You almost have to be a genius to wash your hands before preparing foods properly. So much thought and consideration must take place. It is rocket science to get it perfect. I want perfection in a person who makes my food. Do you believe the employees of the restaurant you choose wash their hands like they are supposed to? I know the answer; everyone knows the answer: ABSOLUTELY NOT!!!

Most of the employees are teenagers or very young adults. They could care less about washing their hands. Some go to work when they are sick. It is a known fact! I'm not paranoid. This is a real problem. You have to understand this fact and know how to defend yourself from unwanted viruses and diseases. The answer is really simple, pick a restaurant that uses gloves. Gloves are intended to remove the need to handle food with your bare hands. Bare hands suck! One small mistake, and your food is contaminated. Wearing gloves and adhering to the strict glove policy (*that includes washing hands before wearing gloves*) is the only defense when young people, or anyone for that matter, are making your food. If someone says washing your hands is perfectly okay to prepare food, why do doctors wash their hands for 5 to 10 minutes and then put protective gloves on before surgery? Let that absorb in for a bit.

The restaurant must have a strict glove-wearing policy. Washing your hands frequently is still a factor. Wearing gloves is not all of it. You also have to be cautious and know when to change your gloves. The more you change gloves, the better the intent will be maintained. Gloves should be replaced when they become soiled or torn, before beginning a new task, every few hours during a continuous task, after handling raw meats, seafood, and poultry, and before and after every sandwich is made. When you do it right, it becomes second nature after a while, meaning you don't even notice the process.

- Explore your options. It is always a good idea to think about nutrition. Most convenience stores like 7-11 or High's have fresh bananas. Grab a banana, a nut-based snack, and water. This is a quick in and out choice when you're in an extreme hurry.

- Never eat at any restaurant that is not crowded with people regardless of the time of day. If that place is not packed with people, turn around and run. There is a reason why it's not busy; it could be bad food, horrible service. Regardless of the reason, their food is most likely old and potentially stale. Always think of the worst case. If you ignore this recommendation, you may be playing with fire; fire out your ass, that is. Don't take that chance!

- Find a restaurant with lots of people; the busier the restaurant, the better. If you have to stand in line for a long time, stand there with a smile. Remember why you picked this place. The more people in the restaurant, the fresher the food will be. I love Jimmy John's and Jersey Mike's. They have a great glove policy and make an awesome sandwich. Those restaurants are always busy, so the food is naturally fresh.

- Avoid restaurants where the food is typically uncovered and exposed. I get a little scared at those places because it's unknown how long the food has been sitting out. But if the restaurant is busy, then the food should be okay. When you place your order, be on the safe side and order a simple sandwich. A ham and cheese sandwich is always a good choice. Avoid veggie-type sandwiches, salads, and lettuce or spinach on your sandwich. There is a very good chance those raw vegetables have not been properly washed. You do not want to be on the road after eating contaminated vegetables with salmonella, listeria, or E. coli. Talk about gastric distress. If this happens, finding a bathroom would not be the prime focus; finding a hospital would be.

- Your last resort would be the heavy, greasy fast-food restaurants. This may work out okay, depending on the menu. Chick-fil-A, in my opinion, is the safest bet. I have never seen a Chick-fil-A not busy. Other places would depend on what foods agree with you.

- You might want to think really hard before you order a pizza unless you made it yourself. Think about the process these pizza restaurants do in making a pizza. You thought it was bad when kids or young adults don't wash their hands properly. What do you think happens at a pizza joint? The entire hand is used in rolling the dough. This means their fingers, fingernails, palms, knuckles, back of the hand, and wrist. Think about that for a second. What do people do when they have an itch or bead of sweat rolling down their face? They use the back of their hand to scratch or wipe up the sweat. The back of the hand is the weapon of choice when your hands are doing something else, like prepping food. What about flipping the pie dough in the air thing? Not only are they mixing hand germs in your pizza dough, let's throw in some arm hair. How often are the arms washed before they make a pizza? I would say NEVER! So, remember, the next time you eat a pizza, think about how it's made, and don't be surprised if you see a few hairs in it. I experienced it. If you're completely honest with yourself, you have too.

- The most difficult thing to remember is never to overeat. This is extremely hard because when you're hungry and factoring in all the time and effort you put into finding the right place to eat, you end up over-ordering. When you are extremely hungry and start to eat, the time it takes from the bag to your stomach is dangerous. Minutes later, you feel bloated and possibly nauseous. There is one fact I guarantee will happen, there will be a bathroom break in your near future. It may not be a pleasant experience either. Always try to eat light and eat small portions throughout the day.

- Be careful with sugar-free sweeteners used in breath mints and chewing gums. The sugar alcohols may cause bloating and diarrhea. This is a huge dilemma for individuals like me who quit smoking cigarettes. Chewing gum is a necessity. Being a hyperactive person is not helping me either. I don't want to have to quit chewing gum as well.

Sugar products will cause teeth to decay, and sugar-free products will put some of us on the toilet. A sugar alcohol called erythritol looks like the best choice for me. According to Wikipedia, erythritol is low in calories, does not affect blood sugar (so a great choice for people with diabetes), does not cause tooth decay, and is less likely to lead to bloating and nausea. Wikipedia states not to consume more than 50 grams per day. That's just fewer than 11 teaspoons. This is when nausea and stomach bloating would occur. In any case, 11 teaspoons of any sugar or sweetener are way too much for anyone to consume in 24 hours.

Try to do some research on the internet at home. See how your picked restaurants prepare their foods, and most importantly, make sure they have a strict glove use policy. I was at a Donut Shop for coffee one day, and the person in front of me ordered a couple of donuts. The employee was already wearing gloves and didn't understand the concept of wearing gloves. She received payment using gloves, gave change using the same gloves, then picked out two donuts using the same gloves, placed the donuts in a bag, and handed them to the customer. She used the same gloves to handle money and the donuts. It never occurred to her to change gloves after playing with money. I didn't say anything at the time because I was shocked. When it was my turn to order, I felt it was my duty to everyone behind me to confront her about this. I asked why she didn't change her gloves after handling money. No response -- just a confused blank stare. I thought I heard crickets in the background. The moral of this story is always to think of a worst-case scenario, be careful in what you order and always keep an eye on the person who is making your food. If you see some shenanigans in making your food, don't be afraid to call them out. Ask for the manager and complain. You have a civic duty to protect those waiting behind you.

There is a lot of anti-bathroom stuff to think about when you're away from home. This may be a trial and error effort in planning your perfect day. Get on the internet and start to educate yourself on the right foods to eat. Make a list of foods you know will not cause you problems, including condiments. Eating healthy, eating fresh foods that agree with you, and remembering to avoid overeating should help those abrupt bathroom challenges throughout your day.

3 PUBLIC BATHROOMS

Before you leave the house each day, create a journey plan similar to a flight plan in what airplane pilots do before they take off from the airport. Map out your entire route for the day and locate several public places along the way with suitable bathrooms.

The most reliable places to stop with semi-clean bathrooms are your large hardware stores such as Home Depot, Lowe's, and most grocery stores. These places typically have several toilet stalls and urinals, so you're almost guaranteed to have a free stall. The riskier places to stop would be your convenience stores such as Wawa, Sheetz, Royal Farms, and other off-road convenience stores. These places are everywhere. The chances of any of these places having clean bathrooms or having toilet paper are under 30%. So always bring toilet paper with you, among other sanitary tools.

Most car dealerships and hotels have nice clean bathrooms. Hotels would be a really good choice because the guests normally use the bathroom in their suite. So, the bathroom in the main lobby will most likely be free. Keep in mind most of these places frown upon anyone using the bathroom if you're not a guest or a guest's friend. But when that time comes and you're running out of options, take the chance. The best approach is to pretend you're picking up a guest at the hotel. Casually walk into the establishment and wander your eyes like you're looking for someone; at the same time, stroll around and slip into the bathroom. When you walk out of the bathroom, continue looking for your friend as you walk towards the exit. Slowly get into your car and drive away. Remember, the bathrooms are provided for guests only, so always be courteous and clean up after yourself. Please don't destroy this option for the rest of us.

Places to avoid are the smaller convenience stores such as 7-11, High's, and most all gas stations. These places typically will not allow public bathroom use. Other bad choices are your fast food joints such as McDonald's, Burger King, Arby's, Pizza Hut, Starbucks, and Dunkin Donuts. These places typically only have one toilet stall, and I will guarantee you somebody will be using it.

One important note, please try and pay it forward. When an establishment allows you to use their bathroom or when a public bathroom is accessible within an establishment, clean up after yourself and report any damage you see or when the toilet paper is empty. Always be kind, respectful, and appreciative. Buy something; it doesn't matter what you buy. Being respectful in this way will help keep the bathroom open for all of us behind you.

The worst places to stop are your highway and interstate "rest areas." You know these places. These places have been established for our convenience to use the bathroom while traveling on state highways. They are the worst! As soon as you get out of your car, you almost smell the urine. There are hundreds of people going in and out of these bathrooms every hour. Think about how much human waste is measured every second. I see people running to the bathroom because they are about to explode. I see the same people running out of the bathroom because of the smell or the condition of the facilities. These places are mostly unstaffed. There is no onsite management or cleaning crew. They are also the hardest places to keep clean and maintained due to high operating costs. If you have no choice but to stop at one of these rest areas, don't be alarmed if the place is a disaster. Chances are something will be wrong, out of place, broken, and unclean. Most definitely, they will be out of toilet paper. If you have to go #2, never sit on the toilet seat. Nothing can clean and disinfect these places properly. Way too much human waste developed in a short time. Do your business and get the hell out as quickly as possible.

What pisses me off is when people purposely urinate on the floor and toilet seat, then wash their hands, throwing the towel on the floor. I've seen teenagers rip towel dispensers off the wall, rip toilet seats off and completely trash the place. The state where these rest areas are placed may not have the proper management to witness or respond when these assholes trash the place. That means the hundreds of people who stop to use the bathroom also have to endure this mess. Sometimes you do not have a choice but to use these bathrooms unless other options are available.

Generally, all public bathrooms, in my opinion, are disgusting. In some cases, you may find a bathroom that appears to be clean. Trust me; it's not clean at all. There are so many things alive inside a bathroom just waiting for someone to enter their ecosystem where you become their feast. I don't care what studies or research say. All public and private bathrooms, in my opinion, are riddled with germs and other potential diseases. I will not be subjected to any of this, and I am sure you feel the same way.

Call me a germophobe, hypochondriac, or freak; I don't care what anyone calls me. I refuse to sit down on a toilet seat and refuse to use a hand blow dryer. I refuse to touch anything inside a public or private bathroom. I am always conscious of my surroundings and extremely careful. I keep a flashlight, hand sanitizer, toilet paper, and many other sanitary tools wherever I go. I am here to tell you there are other clean and safe options to protect you.

Blow dryers are super nasty, riddled with germs and bacteria. Everyone who uses it holds their hands tight up against the grills as the hot air is forced through your fingers. I have to say the hot air on my hands does feel awesome. When you think about it, you begin to realize the reality.

How many kids play with the hand dryer <u>before</u> washing their hands? Think about it for a minute, and please do the research yourself. Examine any cleaning crew while they clean a public or private bathroom. Even the best cleaning crews will <u>NEVER</u> clean the hand blow dryer. They remain un-cleaned for weeks, months, and even years. I bet there are colonies, planets, even solar systems of bacterium inside those things. On the surface, hand dryers seemed like a great idea. You are removing the paper to save the trees, the earth, and the environment, right? That was the initial intent and a good one too. Everyone was installing them; no more paper, and safer too. Hot air to dry hands, perfect. Years later, the research found them riddled with germs and deemed unsafe because there was no effective way to clean them properly. Most establishments who had them went back to paper.

If you suffer from IBS, your window of opportunity in finding a nearby public bathroom just dropped significantly. When I say "window of opportunity," this means you don't have much time to find a toilet before you soil yourself. Many don't understand the concept of what this means for someone with IBS. I am sure most of you may experience this feeling once in a blue moon. But within my IBS family, this may be an hourly occurrence. Like an airplane pilot always looking for a safe place to land in case of an emergency, IBS people constantly locate potential bathrooms along our path. On a good day, my window of opportunity is maybe 15 minutes. On a bad day, under a couple of minutes. So, finding a bathroom for me could be any place I choose. The bathroom I can use or choose to use is never worse than using the Jiffy John or a highway interstate rest area. In my opinion, the state highway rest areas would be the worst experience. But beggars cannot be choosers. So, get it done and be on your way.

Everyone has experienced at some point in their life the uncomfortable feeling of "holding it in." You find yourself desperately trying to find a bathroom as quickly as possible. The longer you wait, the more uncomfortable the feeling becomes. The discomfort moves in waves, and each wave is stronger than the next wave. Soon the discomfort expands into severer pain, anxiety, and sweating. Decisions now become desperate and immediate. You look everywhere for a good place to go, like a trash can, between two cars, behind bushes, etc. At this point, you have very little time to think rationally, and it is all about going, and nothing much in the world matters. If you're in the car, you push your ass cheeks together and turn one way or the other to add more stopping power. When you are on foot, you have to take a knee using the back of your ankle to push it back in. Whatever it takes to get past that wave so you can push on. Seconds feel like minutes and minutes feel like hours. Finally, the moment arrives, and you find a place to go. After you finish up, what an amazing feeling of satisfaction and accomplishment of being able to hold it in long enough to prevent a disaster moment. You experience the overwhelming feeling of comfort, relaxation, and love of God.

When departing the bathroom, you may feel embarrassed if others observed your desperate mission. I don't give it much thought because this is a daily event for me. It is what it is; others know this feeling as well as you do. So put your head down and get the hell out of there. Hopefully, nobody you know witnessed your desperate journey. So, what if they did? Their day will most definitely come.

4 PROCEDURES OF SAFE BATHROOM USE

There are many steps to consider when using a public bathroom. These steps are very important to comprehend to ensure a germ- and disease-free experience. Before you enter a bathroom, you must have an exit plan. Your thought process must be in reverse. Here are some important steps to consider when using a public bathroom.

If someone is in the men's room and you really have to go, use the ladies' room. This is a bold move but sometimes the only choice when your time is running out. Try to get in and out as quickly as possible. I really don't give this much thought because I use the ladies' room all the time. Who really cares what anyone says or thinks? You don't know these people, why should you worry about it? When I get caught, I just smile, apologize and walk away. The manager or customer of the establishment may get upset and throw some words at you, but in reality, they understand why you used it. Again, clean up after yourself, and don't destroy this option for the rest of us.

Make sure you study the surroundings when you walk into a public bathroom. Know where the sinks are located, paper towel dispenser, hand dryers, urinals, and egress. You should also be cautious of what stall or urinal you choose. Don't forget you're in a public bathroom; this means you will not be alone.

Someone may already be inside the bathroom when you enter, and others will come in behind you. Sometimes you have to sacrifice comfort or convenience to protect yourself from all the crazies out there. It is a good idea to carry a compressed air sound horn like the ones used on boats. When you're inside the bathroom, and for some reason you feel threatened or believe shenanigans are afoot, sound the crap out of it. Trust me; they will leave quickly. I would also call 911 immediately to report the incident to protect the next victim.

I always pick a urinal furthest away from the exit door. This way, you will have a direct line of sight showing all obstacles (*including persons*) in your path of travel. If anyone is behind you, that person could potentially whack you on the head and rob you or do something worse. The same choice should be applied when you use a toilet stall; use the one furthest away from the exit door. Typically, this stall would be the handicapped one. I know it's not polite or ethical to use the accessible toilet, but if you know you will be in and out pretty quickly, then safety first.

The reason why you want to use the urinal or toilet furthest away from the exit door is to prevent these wackos from surrounding you. If you're inside the stall door, you can lock the door. If anyone tries to crawl underneath the door, sound the air horn and start stomping your foot on them as hard as you can. If you're standing at a urinal, try to repeatedly kick them in the balls while sounding the air horn. If you're inside the stall and things seem out of place, or you feel uneasy before you unlock the door, look underneath to see where everyone is located. If they are standing by the sink or toilet stall, then things appear to be normal. If they are standing around facing you or standing at odd places, call 911 and sound the air horn immediately. I know this sounds a little panicky, and you're probably right. But I have good reason to feel this way. One of the goals of this guide is to help prevent any harm to you, your family, or friends.

I remember as a kid (maybe six years old) on my way to Hartford, Connecticut, to see my grandmother with my mom and her longtime boyfriend (they never married), to whom I was very close. We stopped at Bob's Big Boy along the New Jersey Turnpike to get something to eat and use the bathroom. As soon as we parked the car, I obviously ran to the bathroom. When I walked into the bathroom, there was this old guy (maybe in his 30s) using the urinal. There were only three urinals, and this guy was using the middle one. I walked up to the urinal to this guy's right because I liked the idea of having the toilet stall door as a barrier. As I was urinating, that old guy was leaning over watching me; I mean actually watching me. His head was turned towards my crotch, with both eyes staring at my penis while I was urinating. I didn't know what the hell was going on. I left the bathroom and found my mom at the table so we could eat lunch. After we finished lunch, I went back to the bathroom again to go one more time because we still had a long way to go on the road. That same old guy was at that same stall and again watching me urinate. I remember feeling extremely uncomfortable and totally creeped out. When I got back to the table, I told my mom and her boyfriend what happened. The boyfriend immediately left the table, saying he had to use the bathroom and would be right back. I had no idea what happened to me in the bathroom or why the boyfriend immediately left the table. What I do know is we had to leave Bob's Big Boy in a really big hurry. There was a lot of commotion and chaos surrounding the men's bathroom. The boyfriend's clothes were all messed up, and he had some blood on his hands. My mom was frantic with tears in her eyes but never said anything to me about what happened and why we were leaving in such a hurry. I have to believe that old guy in the bathroom got the living shit beat out of him, as he should have. My mother never talked about this incident ever. Even when I was well into my 30s, she never told me what happened that day at Bob's Big Boy. Do people really hang out in a public bathroom for sex? Really? Are you serious? You have to be careful not to be put yourself or your children in a position like that one. Prepare your children for the worst-case scenario because there are tons of crazy and sick people in this world.

I strongly recommend the following steps when using a public bathroom. These steps may seem excessive and extremely paranoid, but when you start following them to the letter, you will see how useful and necessary they become.

Step 1: Before you enter the bathroom, examine the entry door to determine how the door will swing when opened. If the door opens into the bathroom, this means you have to touch the door by pulling the handle or turning a knob to exit. In this case, you will need a paper towel, toilet paper, or part of your clothing to exit the bathroom. If the door swings away from the bathroom, all you need to do is push the door open with your arm, foot, back, or shoulder.

Step 2: Once you walk into the bathroom, you need to keep your hands away from your face throughout this entire process. Be extremely careful in what you touch inside any bathroom, even if the bathroom is at your friend's house.

Step 3: Take a visual assessment of the entire bathroom. Evaluate cleanliness, what free stalls are open to use, do the stall doors fully close and latch, do the toilets automatically flush or are they manually operated, is the toilet seat secure, is there plenty of toilet paper, is there plenty of paper towels or do they use hand dryers, is there plenty of hand soap, what type of faucets are in place, are the faucets automatic or manually operated, where is the wastebasket located, what is the distance between the wastebasket and the exit door, is the lighting fixed or on timers. All of this information is extremely important because it requires you to use your hands. You need to plan your exit strategy from the moment you enter the bathroom.

Step 4: Locate the best stall or urinal that is furthest away from the exit door, as discussed earlier in this chapter. Start visually mapping out your exit strategy. Your path of travel will be from the toilet or urinal to the sink to wash your hands, then over to the paper towels so you can dry your hands, then exit the bathroom. Remember the footprint where all these fixtures are located in the bathroom, especially if you are inside a toilet stall. You may need to look under the door to see where everyone is located if you believe something is wrong.

Step 5: Before you sit down, be sure the seat is sturdy and well mounted. The last thing you want is the toilet seat giving way, falling into the toilet bowl or on the floor. I can only imagine what life forms are nesting on the floors and hidden crevasses surrounding a public toilet. If I fell on the floor in a public bathroom, you would need to take me away on a stretcher and medevac me to the nearest psych ward.

I try to tripod whenever possible. But sitting down is much more comfortable, so let's be comfortable. I typically line the toilet seat with toilet paper. This works fine for me; it also provides for a warmer seating experience. I never use those paper toilet seat dispensers. They are way too difficult to use and always a pain in the ass to cover the entire seat properly.

When the seat is properly lined, be careful as you start sitting down. Move slowly until your ass cheeks are placed securely on the seat. If you move too fast, you will create a slight breeze, and the toilet paper will blow off the seat. As you sit down, if you feel something cold on your ass, that means part of you is directly touching the toilet seat. When this happens, it's too late to fix the problem, damage done. Hopefully, you brought hand sanitizer with you to deal with this problem when you're ready to sit up.

Once you are securely seated, start the process of relieving yourself. Remember not to push too hard; let it come out naturally on its own. Pushing too hard may cause an extreme explosion with a devastating splashback. You will not have a nice day if that happens.

If the lighting is on a timer, remember to keep track of time so the lights don't turn off while you're sitting on the toilet. This is why it is important to always have a flashlight on hand. All your smartphones have flashlight apps. If you don't have a flashlight or a smartphone, you're in a lot of trouble; unless you have time to continue sitting on the toilet seat until someone else walks inside. I want out of that place as quickly as possible.

Step 6:   When you finished unloading and cleaned up, time to leave the stall. If your ass was directly touching the toilet seat, use the hand sanitizer and wipe the affected area before pulling up your pants. Buckle up and walk out of the stall. Now it's time to wash your hands. This is one of the most important procedures in this mission. This process may require multiple hand washing.

- If the bathroom has automatic faucet activation, automatic soap dispensers, and automatic paper towel dispensers, this process just got a lot easier. Place your hands under the automatic hand soap dispenser with an excessive amount of soap, place your hands under the faucet and thoroughly wash your hands. Wave your hands under the automatic paper towel dispenser, grasp more than what you need, dry your hands and walk towards the exit door. DO NOT throw away the paper towel just yet; you will need it to exit the bathroom.

- If the bathroom is not equipped with automatic functions, this process will become a little more complicated. If the paper towel dispenser is equipped with a push-down lever type, go to the toilet stall you walked out of and get a small piece of toilet paper you can use to shield yourself from touching the paper towel dispenser lever. Push the lever until 4 inches of paper is hanging, tear the paper off, and throw that part away. Push the towel depressor again until you have a sufficient amount needed to dry your hands. Let the paper towels hang there until after you wash your hands. If the paper towel dispenser requires you to place your hands inside the dispenser to remove the towels, reach inside and remove a sufficient amount. Be sure to take more than what you need. As you pull the towels out of the dispenser, use a clean towel to throw away the first 2 to 4 towels. These towels may be contaminated with remnants or the previous user's remnants. Set aside a couple of paper towels you can use to operate the faucet and hand soap dispenser, secure all the other towels under your arm. Using the paper towel turn the water faucet on and use the hand soap dispenser liberally, then wash your hands thoroughly. Dry your hands with the paper towels secured under your arm or hanging from the towel dispenser. After you dry your hands use the towel to turn off the faucet and walk towards the exit door, do not throw away the paper towels just yet. Remember you need these towels to exit the bathroom.

- If the bathroom is equipped with a hand dryer, <u>NEVER USE IT</u>!!!! The automatic hand dryers are never cleaned. Everyone places their hands tightly under the discharge nozzle; kids play with it without washing their hands. Just stay away from those things! When you have no viable options, use a piece of clothing.

- **Step 7**: As you're walking towards the exit door, hopefully, the wastebasket is open and nearby the exit door. If the wastebasket is open and near the exit door, use the paper towel you used to dry your hands to open the door. Hold the door open with your foot, throw away the paper towel, and exit the bathroom. If the wastebasket is closed or too far away from the exit door, keep it with you and find a place to throw it away later. If the exit door is swinging away from the bathroom, just push the door open with your back or shoulder. Once you leave the bathroom, use the hand sanitizer with liberal amounts as a safety factor. Never use your hands to open the door!!! Trust me, that doorknob or handle will be riddled with germs and diseases.

I know these steps seem obsessive-compulsive, not normal thinking behavior, and even bat shit crazy, but over time you will begin to understand. What appears to be clean is only an optical illusion. If you're not extremely careful, you will eventually expose yourself to diseases, or God knows what else lives inside those public bathrooms.

Practicing safe bathroom use will make you more conscious of potential germs, diseases, and living critters at every corner of the bathroom. Each time you walk into a public bathroom and practice these methods, you will get better and better at it. At some point, a light switch will go off in your head, and you will experience an overwhelming feeling of total awareness and understanding. Eventually, this will become a game each time you use the bathroom. You will also be much more thorough when cleaning your own bathrooms.

Self-awareness is the key to successful clean germ and disease-free bathroom use. Practice makes perfect; perfect bathroom use should be your goal every time.

5 ON THE ROAD AND OUTSIDE

Like the airplane pilot, I am constantly searching for a safe, secluded area to use as a bathroom. When you got to go, you got to go, regardless of where you are. Going outside is where God intended us to go anyway. This is my favorite place because everywhere you look could be a potential bathroom. If you choose to go outside, remember to be courteous to others and not leave anything behind. Just like dog owners, we have to pick up after ourselves. This can be an extremely gross event if you're not prepared for it.

When you're traveling in your vehicle, choices may be limited depending on the window of opportunity. If you have time to pull over to use a safe public bathroom, refer to what we discussed in Chapter 4. When you're on foot, choices are very limited because it is extremely difficult to carry all the items you need in an emergency. I highly recommend purchasing a knapsack and create a bug-out bag. You can put the important toilet essentials you need, such as toilet paper, hand sanitizer, and a poop bag. You can also add life safety items such as bottled water, snacks, a change of underwear (*just in case*), and other stuff you may need. Try not to overstuff your bag. The heavier the bag, the more difficult it will be to travel with it.

We all know pooping outside is filthy. It is also extremely offensive, and if anyone sees you pooping or sees traces of what you left behind, you could be in some trouble. Using this option has to be 100% remnants-free!!! We talk about finding secluded areas using this option later in this chapter.

If you're not pooping directly in a bag and plan on pooping on the ground, you better have some kind of underlayment. After you finish pooping, pick up the underlayment, place it in a bag with your used toilet paper, find a suitable trash can, and discard it. I tried many other options unsuccessfully but was determined to find an easier, cleaner way. One day I used an office trash can bag, and it was perfect. The bag was big enough to fit my entire ass inside. No longer have to worry about aim or precision. Just stuff your ass inside the bag and rip one out. I always carried a few of them with me wherever I went. The only problem is the bag had to be thrown away immediately because of the smell. Now I have the Cleanwaste WAG BAG®- GO Anywhere Toilet Kit® bags that are biodegradable and landfill friendly. Cleanwaste made my life so much easier. I would like to be perfectly clear; I am not affiliated with Cleanwaste in any way. If you lived the past 50 years the way I lived with IBS, you really appreciate it when you find a product that makes your life happier and easier. To leave the house confident knowing you have a suitable bathroom alternative to be more flexible in planning your activities.

Secluded areas are easy to find but usually heavily populated. Trash dumpsters typically have constructed enclosures surrounding the dumpster to hide their appearance. Just slip in behind a dumpster, take care of business, throw it away and move on. The same applies in all other secluded areas you find. In every case, you have to put on some speed. The goal is to get in and out as quickly as possible. It helps if you have a wingman for a lookout. The anxiety of knowing someone could be right around the corner to catch you in the act may slow the process.

The most reliable secluded places are wooded areas. If you're on the road, all you need to do is pull over, hit the flashers on your vehicle, and walk into the woods far enough to shield yourself from other passing cars. The heavier the traffic, the further in the woods you need to go. Make sure you bring toilet paper and a poop bag with you. If you're on a hill, be very careful how you position yourself. When you pull your pants down, they will be at your ankles. Place yourself where your ass is pointing away from your pants. You have to compensate for the steepness of a hill. If you don't compensate, your ass may not be fully in the bag, and you could potentially soil yourself. So be careful...

Depending on where the woods are located, you could bury your poop. In those cases, bring a shovel with you. You can purchase a low-profile shovel at any camping store. They are compactable and easy to travel with. If you choose the bury option, be sure to use white plain unscented toilet paper. You have to be over 200 feet away from wells, ponds, streams, and other waterways. Dig a hole at least 6 inches deep. After you're done, bury it and be on your way. Going to the bathroom in the woods is perfect, peaceful, quiet, and the scenery is spectacular. If this option is in your near future, you may want to educate yourself in the County/State/City rules and procedures in burying poop in your area.

When the window of opportunity is immediate, it's time to pull over wherever you are. If you have a little time, try to find an underpass or bridge. Underpasses and bridges create a shadow from both the sun and the moon, so make sure you park in the shadows. The sunlight and even the moonlight will cause glare to vehicles in your line of sight. Even at night, when headlights shine on you, light is reflected from your rear window or door. If none are near, pull over to the right shoulder as quickly and as safely as possible. I try to place my vehicle in a way to provide more shelter. For example, when you pull over on the right side of the road, the front of your vehicle should be pointing toward 11 o'clock and the rear of the vehicle pointing toward 5 o'clock. Try and find as much camouflage you can between the shoulder of the road and civilization. Hit the flashers, check traffic, get out of the car and walk around to the right side of the vehicle. Open both the front and rear passenger doors, then place yourself right in the middle (*reverse steps for the left shoulder*). If your vehicle has a trunk door, open that door as well. This should provide you with sufficient camouflage to shield yourself from other passing cars.

If you are older having trouble squatting down, you can purchase a portable toilet seat; I use a 5-gallon bucket. If you use a portable toilet seat while in your vehicle, you will be sitting much higher off the ground and preventing natural camouflage. People driving will be able to see you through the car door windows. You may want to purchase two heavy black moving blankets and keep them in the car with you at all times. Just drape the heavy black blankets over each car window. In my opinion, black is the best color regardless of the color of your car. Bright colors will stand out, drawing more attention to what you are doing.

If your vehicle only has one door, your creativeness just got more complicated. In those cases, you can use the camping pull-up tent. The problem with using the pull-up tent is everyone will know exactly what you are doing. They will not actually see you, but they will know what is going on. If you have to use the tent, make sure you pull over under a bridge. I am not a big fan of pull-up tents; those things will blow away on windy days. When you start having problems and using the bathroom becomes more frequent, you may want to purchase a vehicle with a front and back door.

Just throwing out ideas, the goal is to be completely comfortable in the bathroom choice you use and ensure you have the proper camouflage needed to prevent anyone from seeing you. The Cleanwaste WAG BAG®- GO Anywhere Toilet Kit® biodegradable bags will work with most all apparatuses. If you need more options, search the internet. I am sure you will find a solution that will best fit your needs.

6 JIFFY JOHNS

Jiffy Johns are not the cleanest choice. You can pretty much guarantee they are a disaster inside. But when there is nothing in sight, they become your best friend.

We all know what a Jiffy John is. It's another code name for an enclosed portable toilet. These things are four foot squared fiberglass enclosed portable bathroom standing in direct sunlight, limited ventilation, crap piled up close to the toilet seat, and a puddle of piss trapped in the urinal because the drain hole is stuffed with toilet paper. Let's not forget about the hundreds of flies swarming in this small box. Those flies are landing on your body after being knee-deep in crap. For flies, crap is Thanksgiving dinner, and you are their dessert. Just think about this the next time you walk inside one.

I don't care who you are; if you like tailgating, attending outdoor events, or if you work construction, you will have the Jiffy John experience. What's worse is there never seems to be a sufficient amount of Jiffy Johns available for the people who need to use them. You end up standing in line for long periods of time behind many people just waiting and waiting to use one. You can take advantage of the waiting period as an opportunity to prepare yourself for this uncomfortable sequence of events that are about to take place.

In my opinion, the Jiffy Johns are not built for the average person. When you walk in, all you can do is turn in a circle, and there is no room to move forward, backward or sideward. You must have a really good plan of attack. Your plan would need to account for maneuverability and access to your supplies. Make sure you have toilet paper, wet naps, and hand sanitizer. Nose plugs may not be such a bad thing if you plan on spending more than 5 minutes inside. Take off any heavy jackets, sweatshirts, or other layered clothing before you enter. This will help for stable maneuverability. In the summer, you will most likely be wearing shorts and short sleeve shirts, so don't forget about the flies of prey. The best plan is to account for the worst conditions you believe may exist.

Most Jiffy Johns are equipped with hand sanitizer dispensers. Every time I tried to use one, it was empty. I remember being inside one shortly after it was cleaned, and the dispenser was still empty. Do they even refill those things? I am pretty sure the first person to use the Jiffy John after it was cleaned got so grossed out, he or she pumped it dry. You never seem to have enough hand sanitizer to make you feel clean after using one of those things. The only line of defense is your wisdom. To do the best you can to fight whatever landed on you, what you bumped into, and to defend yourself from whatever germs or diseases are inside. Obviously, I am overly inflating the dangers here. My comments are more obsessive-compulsive and germophobic. I'm okay with either. Better be safe than sorry.

The disinfecting blue chemical used in Jiffy Johns is supposed to help stop germs and odor. The smell of this chemical is so overwhelmingly strong you almost cannot go inside. Your eyes will tear, and the smell makes some people sick to their stomachs. I am pretty sure that's not good for you. If you have to use the Jiffy John to take a dump right after it's clean, get ready for some colorful deep blue splashback on your ass cheeks. We talk later in this chapter on how to defend yourself against that problem.

When the chemical color turns green, this means it will no longer help with germs and odors. I am pretty sure everyone reading this guide knows exactly the smell I am referring to after the blue chemical stops working. To paint a picture for those who do not, imagine hundreds of people urinating and pooping inside this four-foot square box with no air freshener or ventilation. Now triple that smell when the temperature outside is above 60 degrees, ten times that smell when the temperature is above 80 degrees. I think you get the picture.

Jiffy Johns are cleaned once a week, every weekend, and before every event. Before you step inside, you have to assume hundreds of people used them before you. One of my biggest fears is having no choice but to use a Jiffy John to take a dump. It's not the deep blue chemical splashback that scares me. It's the hundreds of people before me who urinated and crapped inside mixed all together, splashing back at me. I can't even express in words how disgusting and horrifying that is. I lived this fear for over 50 years. I would have to say at least 75% of my experiences were horrible.

There is no sitting on the toilet seat regardless if you're the first person to use it. The seat paper dispenser or even lining the toilet seat with toilet paper does not help you at all here. The only solution is to place your ass cheeks approximately four inches above the toilet seat using the tripod position. Remember, when using the tripod method, one of your hands will be on the back wall of the Jiffy John, helping to stabilize yourself. Your other hand is needed to prevent the splashback effect. Trust me, when you have that much distance between your ass and whatever mixed liquid horror is below, you will get a significant amount of splashback.

There is no guaranteed method to be splashback-free. You have to go into this knowing you will get some splashback. The heavier the stools, the bigger the splashback, even when you have diarrhea or loose stools. The speed of travel as it expels from your body and when it first hits the liquid below will cause a significant splashback. All you can do is the best you can do to prevent as much splashback as possible.

What I am about to share with you is not a perfect science, but this is what I learned over the past several decades. Before you get into position, ball up some toilet paper into a flat, sturdy consistency roughly six inches square. Make at least 3 or 4 of these shields and place them where you can get to them immediately. Now get into the hovering tripod position and be sure you are stable and comfortable.

Place your hand holding the balled-up toilet paper between the toilet seat and your two legs. Began unloading while positioning the balled-up toilet paper several inches lower than your anus. As the stool drops downward, let it hit the toilet paper as it falls into the liquid below. Do this each time you drop a load. The science here is the toilet paper breaks the fall while directing the splashback towards the inside sides of the toilet. When you have diarrhea or loose stools, this process becomes more difficult. All you can do in this case is to use the balled-up toilet paper as best you can. I am sorry to say, 65% of the time, you will experience splashback on your ass cheeks. Just wipe it off with toilet paper and smother yourself in hand sanitizer or wet naps. Not sure this will help with germs or diseases, but it's all you can do. Try not to think too much about it and go back to the party and enjoy yourself. The damage was done, and you hope for the best.

I know what you're thinking right now. I bet, while reading this chapter, you think you are better than this; much faster and precise. You believe you have the power to unload and pull yourself out of the way to prevent any splashback from hitting you. I'm telling you it's impossible. If it were possible, you would have to be under 25 years of age and faster than lightning. Think about it, you're in a four-foot squared enclosure with little to no maneuverability, and your pants are down to your ankles. The only outcome is you falling over into the urinal, down on the floor, or the splashback will hit other places of your body, including your mouth. Don't get brave or cocky. Be smart, take your time, and be realistic.

Not much to say about proper etiquette here, only to remember the next person to use this box could be your child, a family member, or a close friend. So, try and be courteous to others, and please do not make things worse for everyone else. Aim well for both!!!

7 AT THE BEACH

Most of your public beach places will provide bathrooms. Some places will have a sufficient number of bathrooms, and some places will not. When bathrooms are provided, count on them being Jiffy Johns. Not a bad thing; just plan for it in advance. I spend most of my beach time in Chincoteague Island, Virginia. They provide a sufficient number of bathrooms and are always relatively clean—a great place to spend your vacation, a small beach town with friendly people. I love Chincoteague.

When you arrive at the beach, get your things together and find a place to set up camp. Take a moment to plan your path or travel to the bathroom. What are the ground conditions between you and the bathroom? Will you need shoes? How many people are standing in line? What is the average time for each person inside? You also have to account for assholes. These people use the bathroom to change into their bathing suits or back into their street clothes. If you are one of these people, you're an Asshole!!! Change in the car or at home before you go to the beach. The bathroom is for relieving yourself, and many of us have to go badly, who are in pain, in significant discomfort, ready to blow in our bathing suit. So Please, Get the Out of the Bathroom!

Be prepared when your time comes. Do a dry run and account for conditions along the way. Always keep your shoes in a ready place so you can grab them in a hurry. Don't wait by shortening your window. Get up and make your way to the bathroom soon after you realize you have to go.

Private beaches with public access normally do not provide bathrooms like Ocean City, Maryland. When no bathrooms are available, this is a tough position to be in because beaches are always crowded with people. There are no woods, no suitable secluded areas to hide, just a completely open environment with tons of people surrounding you. In this case, you have to be creative and bold.

When you plan on going to the beach, always wear a bathing suit with no underwear, no matter if you plan on swimming or not. Also, bring a bucket, short camping shovel, toilet paper, poop bag, antiseptic wipes, and hand sanitizer. It is also necessary to have sunglasses, a baseball cap, and a beach towel poncho. The intent is for the poncho to cover your entire body with your head sticking out the center of it. This is necessary for proper cover and maneuverability discussed later in this chapter. You may want to consider making one of these ponchos. It's best to fabricate one out of a beach towel to match the environment you're in. Having these items should be an automatic response regardless of how long you plan on staying on the beach. When nature calls, you have no choice but to respond. In this situation, you may be responding hastily.

Adults on the beach are always wearing sunglasses watching something while lounging in their beach chairs. The sunglasses make it impossible to know exactly what they're looking at. Just because a head is pointed in an obvious direction does not mean they are looking in that direction. If someone is in direct sunlight with their sunglasses off, their eyes will most likely be closed. Otherwise, people may be reading or talking among themselves. They may be watching their children swimming in the ocean or observing attractive men and women walking in the surf. Over 65% of the people on the beach are watching something. Most of their focus is typically in front of them, not what's behind them. Except for young kids, they see and hear everything. These kids are all over the beach playing in the sand, wandering around from family to family, curious about people and other kids surrounding them. Not a good position to be in when that special time comes. When looking for a place to set up camp, try and find a spot where there are fewer people and older kids; it's okay if you have younger kids of your own; it's the other family's kids you should be worried about.

Most beaches have rented houses right on the beach. Some of these houses have pools and may have an outside toilet. On your way to the beach, try and pay attention to see if any of these houses have outside toilets. This is typically never an option, but it doesn't hurt to look around, and you may get lucky. If you happen to find a house with an outside toilet, the people renting the house will most likely never use it because it's outside in the heat and humidity. If someone at the house is outside, in a polite, respectful way, get their attention and very friendly explain to them you're not feeling well. Inquire should an emergency occur if it would be okay if you could use the outside toilet. You will be very surprised by how compassionate others can be. Don't get your hopes up because this option is slim to none. Maybe 1 and 1000 chances this option is open. It doesn't hurt to ask, and it doesn't hurt to look around because you may find a secluded space to use when other options are not available.

Secluded areas are extremely hard to find, but they do exist if you look hard enough. Beach houses are always elevated off the ground to allow for the view of the ocean. Some of these houses have secluded areas underneath them. Look for as many options you can find, study and rate them by best to worst. Map out your paths of travel to each location. Locate a trash can; if one does not exist or is too far away, use a beach house trash can. Remember always looking, always planning.

Taking a leak at the beach is by far the easiest task to complete for both men and women. Most people just walk into the ocean and go. I am not saying that is appropriate, nor do I suggest you do so. Going to the bathroom in the ocean no matter what number is awful and discussing. But guess what? Over 99.99999% of the people on the beach urinate and poop in the ocean. Yep, they all do every single last one of them, including you, even the ones who rented beach houses right on the beach. No one seems to care one bit. Maybe we should at least try to care, not just for the environment but for the courtesy of others. Just because everyone else is using the ocean as a public bathroom doesn't mean we have to. You could pack a suitable gender-friendly apparatus for each of you. When you have to urinate, grab your beach poncho and cover your entire body, slide yourself up the beach chair, uncover your stuff, carefully position the apparatus and go. Do not pack a clear apparatus; no one wants to see what's inside that thing. If you do not have an apparatus and have no choice but to go into the ocean, just do it. In researching the internet, it doesn't define definitively urinating in the ocean as a bad thing.

If either of those options is too difficult, or if you really could care less, use the lazy approach. The ocean is mostly extremely cold, at least for me. In advance, take a bucket over to the surf and fill it up with water. Walk back to your site and set the bucket in direct sunlight, and enjoy the beach. During the day you will be drinking lots of water or adult beverages and that time will surely come. When that time comes, pick up your chair and move away from your party. "Nonchalantly," take the bucket of water that is now warm or even hot and pour some in your lap, saturating your bathing suit. Take a beach towel holding it above your lap, and let it rip. When you're done, move the towel and pour some more water in your lap to rinse off. Stand up and pour the rest of the water, rinsing the chair and sand surrounding the chair below. Take the bucket back to the surf, refill it and place it back in direct sunlight, ready for round two. Move your chair to your original spot and get back to enjoying the beach. Easy-peasy! I know that sounds gross, but you are urinating in your pants anyway when you go into the ocean. You're just bringing the ocean to you, no difference.

Now comes the tough and bold moment when you have to take a dump. If you're at the beach with no public bathrooms like Ocean City, Maryland, take a good look around. Not all of those people on the beach came from the houses or hotels behind you. Most of these people are from the bayside or other areas far away from their rented place. This may be you. Just like we discussed earlier in this chapter, you are aware of your surroundings trying to locate secluded areas you can use to take a dump. Do you really think all these people from the bayside or parked on the street are thinking or searching for the same secluded areas you are in? You'd like to hope so, but chances are they are not. So, if there are no public bathrooms provided and you have to take a dump, where do you think those people are going to do it? The answer is obvious, in the ocean. Where else can they go? This is a crazy, sick, and disease-invested problem found in all beaches with public access.   What if someone's poop washed up in the surf with kids playing? Infants are always putting things they touch in their mouths. I want to throw up just thinking about it. But it's really not these people's fault. Places like Ocean City, Maryland, with public beach access, should take responsibility and provide public bathrooms. So, the next time you are swimming in the ocean, don't be surprised if the SS-POOP crash into you.

Even when public bathrooms are available, there are a lot of other people who take a dump in the ocean anyways. These are lazy, selfish people who refuse to be numeral or respectful to others. These are the same people who ruin our bathroom options by not cleaning up after themselves. I am talking about another class of assholes, the first line of assholes.   These people are easy to spot; they are the ones who are disrespectful to others, who refuse to offer their seat to an elderly or disabled person, who turn their radios screaming loud, who rudely butt in lines, always picking fights, bullies, you know exactly the person I am describing. Real Fricking Assholes!!! If you accidentally set up camp next to or near these people, you better pick up and move immediately. You have to stay far away from these people as possible, protect your family and friends, and always plan to be safe.

When there is no safe, secluded place to go, there are other extremely bold options you can try. These options will be noticed by others but worth the challenge when you're desperate. A shelter can be between two cars, between sand mounds, under rented houses, behind buildings, behind trash dumpsters, or a place on the beach that is not as populated.

Desperate times call for desperate measures.

When good options are exhausted, worst case and last resort options are now in play. Whatever place you can find may not be foolproof; there is a very good chance someone will see you. Find the most private place you can with as much cover as possible. Hopefully, you will find a corner wall so all your focus will be in front of you and not behind you. If anyone sees you, try not to pay too much attention to them and look the other way. The hat and sunglasses will provide a disguise, and if anyone is looking directly at you, it will appear you do not see them. This may help divert attention away from you. Nothing to see here! It is very important to be 100% ready to go before beginning the process. Spot your place, study your exit strategy and locate the nearest trash can. This is a drop-and-go option, so make sure you're wearing a beach poncho, you have plenty of toilet paper, and your poop bag is ready. When the coast is as clear or as clear as possible, as quickly as humanly possible, drop your pants, slump down, poop in the bag, clean up, stand up pulling up your pants, and place the poop bag in the storage bag. Quickly get the hell out of there and throw away the poop bag. Before you go back to your family or spot on the beach, take a seat someplace and observe everyone around you. Make sure no one is paying attention to you. It is possible someone saw you and be upset or even call the police. You don't want that drama around your family or friends. As long as you did everything you could to shield yourself and did not leave any evidence, I doubt anyone would call the cops. When everything seems normal, take off your beach poncho and make your way back to your beach site.

Here is a great option to practice. Dump your bucket of water and pre-line the bucket with your poop bag. Put your beach poncho on and wear your baseball cap and sunglasses. Hide your toilet paper and hand sanitizer under the poncho. Find a remote, unpopulated and secluded area. Set the bucket on the ground and take a seat, and pretend you're just sitting there passing the time. Initially, people will be looking and curious about what you're doing, but they will lose interest quickly. When you feel most of the people in your line of sight are not paying attention to you, slowly pick yourself up, pull down your bathing suit and sit back on the bucket, do your business, clean up, slowly pick yourself up, slip your bathing suit back on, pull the poop bag out of the bucket and sit back down on the bucket. Quickly place the poop bag into the storage bag and liberally use your hand sanitizer. Look around for a trash can. When spotted, stand up holding the poop bag under the poncho, and pick up the bucket. Throw away the poop bag and get back to the beach site. This option will take plenty of practice to get right. The poncho works great in these situations, with instant cover with no effort. So many tasks can be hidden under the poncho. When this option is done correctly, no one will ever know what you're doing.

When there are no other options to consider, I guess you have to be one of those assholes and go into the ocean. This really sucks. Damn you for considering it. But this is the very last option other than going in your pants. What else can you do when the beach provider does not provide public bathrooms. When you got to go, you got to go! Your last and only option would be in the ocean. The best approach is to start your reconnaissance in the early stages. Locate areas in the water with as few people as possible. Make sure you swim out away from shore to a safe distant location. Be conscious of riptides. You may want to educate yourself on this subject to protect yourself and your family. Riptides are very dangerous and common. Also, check tides, praying you're in an outgoing tide when you have to go. If you drop a load in an incoming tide, watch out, little Johnny. The tide will eventually take your poop to shore. You know how curious kids are. They will pick it up, thinking it's a sea creature, and take it back to their parents, asking Mom, Dad, what's this? These are the chances you have to take when the beach provider does not provide public bathrooms. So, if little Johnny finds a brown torpedo, you don't want anyone to know who launched it.

When you plan your vacation, research the beaches to make sure they provide public bathrooms. If they have public bathrooms, check feedback on the internet. If the bathrooms are disgusting or maybe not enough of them, I am sure someone will report it. The best vacation plan is based on research. If the beaches you want to vacation on do not provide public bathrooms, choose another beach place. In every case, choose a place you and your family will be safe, comfortable, and most importantly, clean. Protect your family and choose wisely.

8 ON A BOAT

Boating is a passion I've had my entire life. I live on the Chesapeake Bay near Deale, Maryland. During the warmer months, that's where you'll find me. I am also a huge fan of Chincoteague Island in Virginia. I try to spend as much time there as possible. The fishing in Chincoteague is awesome; the flounder is all over the place. Depending on the weather conditions, I navigate my boat in the Atlantic Ocean to Black Fish and other artificial reefs. Being out in the ocean is so peaceful, beautiful, and a lot of fun.

.

My uncle owned a 42-foot sailboat with sleeping quarters, a small kitchen, and a toilet. He was a Navy Captain and retired as an Armorial. He took my two older brothers and me on a day trip to St. Michaels, Maryland, across the bay from Annapolis, Maryland. On our way to St. Michaels, I used the bathroom several times. I was having a bad day and clogged the toilet. As he was unclogging the toilet, my uncle said, "*You must have used 40 yards of toilet paper.*" He physically pulled out all the toilet paper I used out of the toilet with his bare hands. It was so gross, and he was so pissed. I felt terrible and embarrassed. In my defense, he knew I suffered from IBS and never schooled me on how to use the toilet properly. But I was not going to defend myself because his hands were literally covered in my shit, so my bad.

On our way back from St. Michaels, the Chesapeake Bay started to get out of control. Out of nowhere, we were caught in the early stages of Hurricane Agnes. This was back in 1972, and I was only ten years old. In the center of the cuddy cabin below deck, there was a table that folded down. In the middle of the table was the sail mask. I remember sitting in the middle of the folded-down table with my arms around the mask, holding on for dear life. The boat was literally sideways, waves were crashing inside the boat, and stuff was flying all over the place. I am not sure what was happening on deck, but I heard a lot of yelling from my uncle, ordering my older brother to respond to tasks he did not know how to perform. It was basically the definition of a "clusterfuck." My other brother was sitting on the steps holding on to the stair rail with a death grip. We both looked at each other in tears knowing we were going to die and no way we would survive this. But we did.

When we finally docked the boat, I remember my uncle sitting on a bench holding his head with both his hands. Here is a guy with 30 years in the Navy and 20 years as a Navy Captain. I would have to say he was the most qualified sailor on the bay. He didn't say anything to us at the time, but many years later, he told us that day was the most scared he has ever been. If we were with any other captain, none of us would have survived. We never went sailing again. Maybe it was the 40 yards of toilet paper with shit hands, or maybe we were just too scared to take the chance. What I do know is this is one memory none of us will ever forget.

If you're on a boat, depending on the size of the boat, it can be extremely challenging when you need to go to the bathroom. Larger boats typically have a head (*toilet*). Many years ago, toilets were called heads in sailing ships. The toilet was placed in the boat's bow with vents and slots cut near the floor, allowing waves crashing into the boat to rinse and wash out the toilet. The captain of the ship used a private toilet typically placed in the stern of the boat. Today they still call them heads, but they are toilets just the same. These toilets will have special operating procedures.

Not all toilets on a boat operate in the same manner. Before you use the toilet, discuss operations procedures with the captain of the boat. This is a lesson I learned abruptly as a ten-year-old kid. Smaller boats do not have toilets, so you need to improvise.

When you're on a boat without a head or toilet, and you have to go, almost 99% of you look to the water. That is a normal response, and all of you are 99% accurate. It does not mean you have to be one of those people. The Cleanwaste WAG BAG®- GO Anywhere Toilet Kit® biodegradable bags and portable toilet seat would be perfect for small boats. The portable toilet can be easily stored and takes up very little room. Used poop bags need to be stored in a suitable closed container. You never know how long you will be on the water. Those bags will start to smell pretty bad after a short while. Don't forget to bring your beach poncho for cover.

If you're on someone else's boat without your bug-out bag and no portable toilet, I guess you have no choice but to go in the water. When you have to go, you have no choice but to choose: go in the water or go in your suit. When you really think about it, water creatures piss and shit in the water, so why can't we. It's not like fish or other water creatures constructed public bathrooms for themselves. I don't claim to be a scientist or marine biologist, nor do I have the necessary knowledge or experience to know exactly what would happen if anyone released human waste into the water. But what the hell else are we supposed to do when there are no other options? I want to be an environmentalist and will always try my best to do my part. All of that sounds perfect until you have to take a shit! I wonder if human waste could be considered organic and fertilizer for marine plants. It would sound so much better if that were true, but we all know it's not. So, if you're an environmentalist or activist who is against anyone pooping or peeing in the water, stay at home. You are a buzzkill, and no one wants you on board. One way or another, Mother Nature will respond. You can't stop it!

Before you board a boat, always discuss bathroom breaks with the captain before you shove off. If the captain says you would need to go in the water or use a portable toilet and you refuse to do so, you better get off the boat. The captain <u>will not</u> attempt to navigate his or her boat to dry land so you can use a proper toilet. Not going to happen!

There are no practical methods you can apply on a boat. Boats are floating on top of the water and move with the current, wind, and wakes from other boats. This is not a stable environment, and movement is unpredictable and can be extremely significant. No conscious person should attempt to try and poop in a container or poop bag without sitting down on something stable. Even if you tried, no one is that good! There is an 85% chance you will fail. If you do try, count on having crap on your hands, clothes, and even the boat. When a strong wake hits, shit will fling everywhere like a scared monkey. Everyone will have to endure the smell for the rest of the trip, and <u>YOU'RE</u> the person to blame. The moral of this story, listen to your captain and do exactly what he or she tells you to do. The captain is responsible for everyone on the boat. If you have a problem with that, don't board the boat.

On a typical boating day, there should not be many people swimming in the water. You may see some water skiing, but for the most part, it should be pretty clear. If there are people in the water, have the captain navigate to a more secluded and private place. Here are a few options you can practice. The most common option is to jump overboard and go. You may have to remove your suit depending on what number, but this can be an easy process. When you have to go #1, most guys can lean over the side of the boat. Gals mostly use the stern ladder dipping their buts in the water to go. But when #2 is afoot, and poop bags are not an option, in the water, you must go. Grab some antiseptic biodegradable wipes and give them to someone on the boat to hold for you. Before you jump into the water, study your surroundings. In tidal waters, see what way the current is pulling you. This is extremely important because after you go, you don't want to float into it. Swim away from the boat for privacy, pull your swimsuit off and go. Now for the gross and discussing task, you have no choice but to endure the wiping of your ass process. You really do not have many options here. You can't use toilet paper, and you can't technically use wipes because of the environment. Yep, you guessed it: you have no choice but to use your hand and fingers to wipe the remnants off your ass and cheeks. After you clean up, well, clean up is not exactly accurate in this case, but as clean as it gets, put your bathing suit back on and swim as fast as you can against the current or away from where you were. When you're at the boat, have the person you entrusted to hold the biodegradable wipes throw them to you while you're still floating in the water; make sure they are pre-opened. Wipe your hands thoroughly, and then climb back into the boat. When you're back on board, use the antiseptic wipes again and smother your hands in hand sanitizer. Lastly, forget about what just happened and get on with it.

I always keep a 5-gallon bucket on my boat just in case. I use the 5-gallon bucket as my portable toilet seat. But when you have no poop bags on the boat, you can use the bucket as a manual toilet. Using the bucket method is very easy. Lean over the boat to capture some water in the bucket, about 3 inches of standing water will be sufficient. If other people are on the boat, go to the stern of the boat and ask everyone else to go to the bow of the boat facing away from you. Put on the beach poncho, knee or sit down on the bucket and go. Place the toilet paper in a suitable closed container or bag, empty the bucket into the water, rinse out the bucket thoroughly and you're on your way.

It gets tricky when other people are on the boat. It's even trickier when your boat is surrounded by many other boats. As a boat captain, you need to instruct your passengers to alert you in the early stages of using the bathroom. Then, when someone says they have to use the bathroom, the captain can immediately navigate the boat to a safe and secluded area as quickly as possible. If you don't have time to navigate to a safe place, the bucket is the best and safest play using the beach poncho.

Funny story: when I was a kid, my cousin, who was much older, rented a 13 ½ foot Boston Whaler and took my brothers and me out on the bay in Ocean City, Maryland. This must have been about 1970 something. Too far back to know exactly how old I was. We were cruising around having a blast, and my cousin had to take a dump. We were in the middle of the bay, so it was obvious what he was going to do. He stopped the boat, jumped into the water, and grunted one out. This huge torpedo shot out of the water right in front of him. Immediately after this happened, a seagull flew down, scooped it up, and flew away. I couldn't believe what I was seeing. This seagull was flying away with this piece of crap hanging out of both sides of his beak, thinking he scored the motherload. This was one of the funniest moments of my life, and we all laughed so fricking hard. I will never forget that day.

9 DROP AND GO

If you are considering this option, it must be too late to find a secluded area or suitable place to go to the bathroom. Right now, an immediate decision is going to be made because you are seconds away from blowing in your pants. In this option, there is no time for wiping, hence the phrase "Drop and Go." Being courteous in this case is not always in your mission plan. You have one goal, and that is to get this hell out of your body immediately. Try and find any place with as much cover as possible, between two cars, in bushes, or maybe a corner of anyplace. Even a crowd of people could be considered cover, depending on the circumstances.

In this option, you have no choice but to poop directly in the bag anyplace you can. The goal here is for this process to be accomplished in seconds. Whatever you can do to shave off some time, you must plan to do it. While looking for a spot, start getting ready. Remove or rearrange clothing. If you have any items that you're holding or carrying, secure them. Take your poop bag out of the package and arrange it in a ready position. Ball up a huge wad of toilet paper and place it under your arm. Remember to try and remain calm and pay attention to every detail. Keep in mind your pants will be dropped to your ankles, so make sure the poop bag and wad of toilet paper are readily accessible. If you're out of sync just a little bit, things will get messy. This will be happening extremely fast. Just do the best you can. Don't think about anything else other than your mission. Find your spot and stand ready.

It's time. When the coast is as clear as it's going to get, drop your pants, place the poop bag under the drop zone, unload, place the balled up toilet paper between your ass cheeks, pull up your pants, and get the hell out of there as fast as you can. Don't stop regardless of who may be screaming behind you. As you are running, always keep your head facing downward and throw away the poop bag in the first trash can you see. When you feel the coast is clear, stop running and find a normal bathroom or secluded area you can use to clean up properly. The balled-up toilet paper should help prevent soling of your underwear and pants. Not a perfect science, but the alternative is much worse. I'll take my chances.

The Drop and Go option should be <u>next</u> to your last resort. People will see you and may even take a picture or video with their phone using this option. Everything these days is uploaded on social media. Chances are it will go viral, and everyone will see it. Can you imagine the embarrassment and humiliation if they knew it was you in the video or picture? If your boss knows it was you, you may get fired. So many bad things could happen using this method. So always keep your head down and <u>NEVER LOOK UP</u>!!! You don't want anyone to know who that person was who took a dump in a bag.

If you choose the Drop and Go option, remember to keep your head down and time is of the essence. Depending on the situation, Drop and Go typically takes between 8 to 12 seconds from pants unbuckle to pants re-buckle. This is assuming you have to go so bad it will explode out of your anus when you give the go code. If you're constipated, I am pretty sure you have the time to find a suitable bathroom because you're all plugged up.

Now you have the <u>very last option</u>, which is to blow in your pants. If this happens, your day is done, just go home, hose off and blow off the rest of the day. This is protocol; trust me, everyone understands.

If you ever have to Drop and Go, God Bless You. I feel your pain and completely understand why you used it. I am also sure you considered the repercussions that could potentially happen using this option. You made a choice and believed it was the only choice. You were in a bad place. But here is something else to think about. It was obviously an emergency. There was no controlling the expelling force of nature. You responded to a process every human being experiences. Unfortunately, your body chose that specific time and place to begin that hateful event. Yep, you pulled your pants down to poop in public. But you did try to conceal yourself as best as you could. You also bagged your poop and threw it away in a trashcan. In my opinion, you did everything within your power to be as civil as possible. You also did not leave any remnants behind. Due to things beyond your control, I believe you responded as decently as a human being could.

When people walk their dogs, does anyone think to place an underlayment under the dog's anus before it poops? When you pick up the dog poop and bag it, how many remnants are left behind? The answer is "lots of remnants are left behind." What do people do with the poop bag? They throw it away in the trash can. Do they use biodegradable bags? Most people do not.

I believe humans should be able to poop outside just like pets. If you're really good at it, no one will ever know you did. You did the best you could to deal with a situation you had no control over, the way I see it. If you get caught by Johnny Law, you will most likely be arrested for indecent exposure. If this happens, you better have tried to conceal yourself and not leave anything behind. If you screwed up even a little, the law would hurt you way more than just blowing in your pants. Sometimes blowing in your pants is the option, whether you like it or not. Shit Happens!!! Deal with it and move on.

10 PORTABLE BATHROOMS

When you're no longer able to maneuver freely or squat down safely, you must have a stable option that is easy and quick to set up. There are so many portable toilets on the market today you can choose from. The best place to shop for portable toilets is your outdoor camping store. My favorite is the five-gallon bucket. This will be a great option if it works for you. I bet you have at least two or three buckets in your garage right now. The bucket also has many uses and is incognito to its primary function. The Cleanwaste portable toilet seats are also another great choice. It folds up and easy to store. The Cleanwaste WAG BAG®- GO Anywhere Toilet Kit® biodegradable bags will work with most all portable toilets, even the five-gallon bucket. When you leave your home, it may be a while before you can use a public or private bathroom. Everyone should consider having a Plan B. You should have a portable toilet or stable method for going to the bathroom in your vehicle at all times. Depending on the circumstances, you may need to sit down once in a while.

Using the portable toilet in public cover becomes more difficult and could be time-consuming depending on your cover method. Camping stores carry simple pull-up tents that can set up in seconds, lightweight, and easy to store. When using the tent, everyone will know exactly what you are doing, and on windy days, the tent may be difficult to set up and keep in place. Just be careful and find a way to secure the tenant properly.

Frankly, I do not care what people assume I am doing as long as they do not see what I am doing. People like me don't have much time to set up cover. I may have seconds to respond. I believe everyone should be thinking along those lines when creating cover in the fastest amount of time.

What would be the fastest cover to set up and easily stored? This is a great question, and it may take a while to figure it out. Bring your family and friends together and crowdsource many good ideas. Whatever you fabricate must be quick to set up, lightweight, and easily stored. I believe the best choice is to take advantage of what is already in place, like sitting right between your vehicle's front and rear doors. I open both doors and drape two heavy moving blankets over them. If it's a windy day, I roll down the window a bit and place the end of the blanket through the open window, then close the window. I place my five-gallon bucket right between the doors, insert the poop bag, sit down and unload. The distance between the two doors may be tricky to pull off. I'm a pretty thin guy, and this works for me just fine. I am sure you will find a method that works for you. When it is time to go, follow the procedures discussed in the "On the Road and Outside" chapter to pull over on the side of the road safely.

When I get to the age when I'm no longer able to maneuver freely or squat down safely, I'm going to be in a lot of trouble. I may invest in a mini motorhome - it seems like a good idea. At some point, adult diapers will become a reality. I am pretty sure adult diapers are in my near future. Maybe this is not a bad thing for me or anyone. When you get to that age, you have to keep an open mind. Yes, they are gross and disgusting, but it will get out of the house. Go wherever you want, drop a load whenever you want. You could have fun with it. Hey Johnny, pull my finger? Then there is the smell, and you cannot hide that. What are you going to do, stay at home until you're dead? You have a valid excuse; you're old. If anyone has a problem with the smell, they can stand somewhere else. The point is to continue living until your time comes. Don't worry about everyone else; you be you and let them be them.

There will be a point in your life when you require assistance. Life sucks hard when you reach the age of dependence, and the assistance of others becomes a reality, the true definition of the circle of life. You come into this world dependent on your parents to take care of you, change your diapers, feed, and take care of you. Then you get old, and your kids or some other poor soul has to take care of you in the same way. This moment is the most humiliating you will ever experience during your entire lifespan. You will be overwhelmed, embarrassed, and humiliated because you have no choice but to lie there, unable to resist or react. Fully aware and conscious observing your children's process and facial expressions changing your diaper, wiping your ass, cleaning your private parts of your body, and trying to feed you. All you can do is exist and witness the horror of being useless. Just like when you were a baby, except a baby can move and react to unpleasant events. Death seems more desirable and necessary. Just thinking about it pisses me off. I am not sure I want to live that long to experience it for myself.

11 CLOSING REMARKS

Food and water are considered fuel and must be consumed to survive. Eating and drinking can be heavenly, so good, that people get addicted to them. However, if you're not careful, food can also harm you. Remember, whatever goes in must come out. Will it come out easy and painless, or will it come out on fire, painful, messy, and explosive? The answer can be easy. What did you eat? How much did you eat? How fast did you eat it? How much stress and anxiety are you under? We all know the first one, but the second, third and fourth are very important. They all work together. Everyone experiences stress and anxiety in one fashion or another, and some days can be overwhelming. Stress and anxiety may cause overactivity in your gut, and when combined with poor food choices, well, I guess you can predict the outcome. Everyone deals with stress and anxiety differently. Life can be very hard, and stress and anxiety are sometimes unavoidable. If you suffer from excessive stress and anxiety, please discuss this with your doctor. When not treated in the early stages, excessive stress and anxiety can cause other health problems.

Eating too much food requires your organs to work harder. They secrete extra hormones and enzymes to break the food down. To break down food, the stomach produces hydrochloric acid. If you overeat, this acid may back up into the esophagus resulting in heartburn.

Meals that are too large or high in fat, coffee, caffeine, or alcohol may provoke abdominal cramps and diarrhea symptoms. Eating too much of some types of sugar that are poorly digested by the bowel can also cause cramping or diarrhea.

You should eat slowly and chew your food. Food needs to break down until it loses texture. It's recommended you chew about 32 times before you swallow. Eating too fast increases the risk of becoming overweight and is linked to a higher risk of insulin resistance, characterized by high blood sugar and insulin levels. It also causes Dumping Syndrome, a rapid gastric emptying because the contents of the stomach empty too quickly into the small intestine. Eating can trigger symptoms such as diarrhea, especially eating meals with high sugar content. Because the food is passing through your intestines so quickly, they might not be able to keep up, and the air mixed with the food can cause bloating, cramping, diarrhea, or vomiting in some cases. When you eat too fast, you swallow more air, which can cause bloating and gas. Slowing down and properly chewing your food helps break down larger food particles into smaller ones, aiding digestion. Please eat well and healthy and take care of yourself.

I wonder if science or evolution will one day resolve how the body reacts to certain foods. To allow all humans to eat or drink whatever they want and never get fat, never get sick, and never have to experience the pain of unloading. Maybe they will invent a human vaporizing digestive system; how awesome that would be. Eat and drink what you want; your body absorbs what it needs, then the rest is vaporized. The vapor would have to be expelled from your body, so why not add a delightful smell feature? Also, it would need to be expelled in someplace other than your anus unless farting is part of the new society and encouraged. What a perfect world it would be. Eat and drink whatever I want and expelling lemony fresh rips. Wow, perfect. I guess I was born too early.

This is another freak of nature. Earth is a violent planet. Every living creature, including human beings, has to kill to survive. Animals killing other animals for food, fish killing other fish for food, and humans killing everything they see for food. Even plants absorb sunlight and water to survive, and some plants eat other living things. It seems like everything on this planet has to murder something or someone to survive. This is God's will. Not only did God make all living creatures murderers and savages, but He also gave all of us the gift of untimed, unscheduled, painful waste removal. Thanks, God!!!

Human survival is remarkable and interesting. Maybe God intended us to be savages. The only information we have from God is a book written by man. Who really knows what is true or what is fabricated? In my opinion, I believe the Bible was created to scare us into a way of life we really do not understand. It's almost controlling for the weak-minded. What the church cannot defend, they say we must have faith. God has a plan; God works in mysterious ways. I believe God chooses not to be in control, to allow us to choose for ourselves and allow this earth to unwind accordingly. I also believe God is not perfect. There are too many ungodly inhuman events happening on this planet to have faith. Just turn on the TV, read a newspaper or listen to the radio. All you hear and see are murderers, rapists, human traffickers, drugs, vandalism, politics, so much evil in this world. If God were perfect, we wouldn't have cancer, Parkinson's, multiple sclerosis, birth disabilities, Irritable Bowel Syndrome, and many other diseases. If God were perfect, there would be no diseases, no hate, no crime, and no defects. The human brain would be perfectly aligned where each of us shares the same love and choose to live in harmony. The gift of being a better person, furthering our education, being nice and considerate to others, having a positive impact on life and this planet, thankful for the gift of life, and helping preserve it. I personally believe there is more evil in this world than good. I hope one day this will change.

I also believe God did not predict his creations to be living in heavily populated cities such as New York, Chicago, or Los Angeles. If you believe in the Bible, Adam and Eve were the first humans. Even if you don't believe in the Bible, whoever placed us here, whatever we spawned from, if we descended from apes, aliens dropped off, abandoned, or however we got here, there were no cities, no buildings, no roads, only openness of nature. Bathrooms in that time would be any place you choose at any time you want. Just squat and go. Now, this makes sense; human beings were meant to expel waste anywhere and anytime they choose.

Regardless of the problems we live in today, life is a privilege no matter what hand you are dealt. When I was a child, my mother told me there is always someone else much worse off than me. I remember as a child sitting on the toilet in severe pain, tears pouring out of my eyes screaming bloody murder, "Make it Stop!!! Make it Stop!!!" My mother walked into the bathroom to care for me and pulled out a National Geographic magazine. She showed me pictures of adults and children around the world who are suffering from hunger, diseases, living in huts or structures made from trash and debris, children with stomachs enlarged by hunger, and it was horrifying. But every time I was sick or experiencing a painful episode on the toilet, I think about what those people have to go through every day. How fortunate I am in body and mind. It could be worse; I could be them.

We are human beings, and we are not perfect. We are what God made us. We do not have to ability to override what our bodies put into motion. It is also understood society does not provide us a sufficient number of public bathrooms placed at various locations surrounding our travel. So, we as human beings have to compensate by locating other resources to use as a bathroom. Whatever bathroom you choose, regardless if it is outside or inside in a public restroom, you have to be courteous to clean up after yourself. Poop into a biodegradable bag and place it in the trash. Make sure you flush and don't leave a clogged toilet. If you do clog the toilet, tell the manager or supervisor; just don't leave. Make sure the bathroom, public, private, or outside is better than when you entered. You could very well be the next person to use this bathroom, so again don't ruin it for all of us.

When you're using the bathroom outside or places not designed for public use, keep in mind this is technically against the law. If you get caught by anyone, including the police, the simple answer is nature called, and there are no safe, convenient or suitable public bathrooms for you to use. This is an uncontrollable human occurrence that is not timed or scheduled. You had no choice but to respond to this uncontrollable event, and you responded to the best of your abilities. You were also being environmentally conscious by cleaning up after yourself. As long as you are courteous, provide proper cover not to expose yourself to others, and clean up after yourself, I doubt very seriously the judge will charge you. In fact, the judge may applaud you. If you're good at this, you will never get caught. I've been doing this for over 50 years successfully.

I hope I could help you deal with this problem more open-mindedly; you are just like everyone else. We are who we are, and going to the bathroom is part of life. Why should we be prudent as to where we go? Why should we only use what society says we have to use? As far as I am concerned, I will go just about anywhere regardless of what people say. As long as I clean up after myself, they can all screw themselves. Who cares what these jackasses think anyway?

Final recap: Depending on your day-to-day schedule, always remember to keep on hand a flashlight, hand sanitizer, antiseptic wipes, toilet paper, a biodegradable poop bag, beach poncho, and whatever else you will need during the course of the day. Start your bug-out bag, and make sure you carry it with you everywhere you go. Be creative and always have an open mind. Be aware of your surroundings and always study everything. Cover is by far the most important part of this process.

Life is great; make it even better. Practice this guide, knowing you no longer have to drive all over creation to find a suitable bathroom anymore. You no longer have to wait in long lines to relieve yourself anymore. You no longer have to endure disgusting disease-infested public bathrooms anymore. This is not rocket science, and you can do this. Practice makes perfect. The more you practice, the better life you have. Enjoy yourself and don't be afraid to leave your house. Grab your bug-out bag and be on your way. Always be kind, respectful, caring, and help anyone you can. Be a good person, and don't be afraid to take chances.

I hope this guide has helped you become more open-minded when it comes to going to the bathroom. Using a public or private bathroom must always be your first choice. But when that time comes, and there are no bathrooms in sight, well, you now have a plan B, C, D……

Live Well, and God Bless You. Have a Wonderful and Safe Life!!!!!!

www.ingramcontent.com/pod-product-compliance
Lightning Source LLC
Chambersburg PA
CBHW071124030426
42336CB00013BA/2191